SILENT WARRIORS

THE YOUTH CANCER ENIGMA

Uncovering Trends, Advocating Awareness, and Igniting Hope for a Cancer-Free Tomorrow

Dr. S.J. Bennett

Table of Contents

Introduction

In the quiet corners of hospitals, amidst the bustling streets of our cities, and within the depths of our communities, a silent battle rages on. It's a battle fought not by seasoned warriors clad in armor, but by the youth of our generation—unexpected soldiers in a war they never imagined they'd face.

Picture this: a vibrant 30-year-old, full of life's promise, suddenly confronted with a diagnosis that shatters their world. Cancer. It's a word that echoes with fear, uncertainty, and a sense of injustice. Yet, increasingly, it's a reality that young people across the globe are forced to confront, defying the assumptions of age and vitality.

The rise in cancer incidence among the youth is not just a statistic; it's a stark wake-up call to the urgency of our times. From bustling metropolises to serene rural landscapes, the youth cancer enigma has woven its tendrils into the fabric of our society, leaving a trail of questions in its wake. Why are more young people succumbing to this relentless adversary? What unseen forces are driving this alarming trend? And most importantly, what can we do to turn the tide?

In the pages that follow, we embark on a journey—a journey of discovery, of empathy, and of unwavering hope. "Silent Warriors: The Youth Cancer Enigma" is not just another book; it's a call to arms, a rallying cry for change in the face of adversity. Through the stories of those touched by cancer, the insights of medical experts, and the collective wisdom of advocates, we aim to unravel the mysteries of the youth cancer epidemic.

Our mission is clear: to shed light on the shadows of silence, to amplify the voices of the unheard, and to ignite a beacon of hope for a future free from the grip of cancer. As we delve into the depths of this enigma, let us stand united in our resolve, for it is only by facing the darkness that we can truly appreciate the light.

So, dear reader, brace yourself for a journey unlike any other. Prepare to be inspired, challenged, and moved to action. For in the heart of adversity lies the seed of resilience, and in the unity of purpose lies the power to change the world.

Welcome to "Silent Warriors: The Youth Cancer Enigma." Let the journey begin.

Chapter 1

Understanding the Surge

In the dimly lit corridors of hospital wards, where the hushed whispers of concern mingle with the beeping of machines, a silent epidemic is unfolding. It's a phenomenon that defies the bounds of age and vitality, casting its shadow over the lives of young adults with alarming frequency.

As we navigate the labyrinth of statistical data and trends, a troubling picture begins to emerge. The once reassuring notion of youth as a shield against the ravages of illness is shattered, replaced by a stark reality: cancer is no longer an affliction reserved for the elderly. Instead, it's encroaching upon the lives of the young with a relentless fervor.

Across the globe, from bustling urban centers to serene rural landscapes, the youth cancer surge knows no bounds. It manifests in various forms, each more insidious than the last. Breast cancer, once thought to be a disease of older women, now claims the lives of young mothers and daughters. Colorectal cancer, typically associated with age and lifestyle choices, is on the rise among those in the prime of their lives. And the list goes on, with each type of cancer leaving its indelible mark on the youth demographic.

But what lies at the heart of this unsettling trend? What forces are at play, driving the surge in youth cancer rates? It's a question that demands answers, and one that we cannot afford to ignore.

Geographical disparities offer a glimpse into the complex web of factors contributing to the rise of youth cancer. In regions where access to healthcare is limited and environmental pollutants run rampant, young adults are disproportionately affected by the scourge of cancer. Yet, even in affluent societies, where healthcare resources abound and public awareness is high, the youth cancer epidemic persists, serving as a sobering reminder of the indiscriminate nature of this disease.

Lifestyle choices, too, play a significant role in shaping the landscape of youth cancer. Sedentary habits, poor dietary choices, and environmental toxins all contribute to the heightened risk faced by young adults. In a world where convenience often trump's health consciousness, the consequences of our actions are felt most acutely by those least equipped to bear them.

But amidst the darkness, there is a glimmer of hope—a beacon of resilience that shines bright in the face of adversity. For every statistic, there is a story of courage. For every diagnosis, there is a community of support. And for every challenge, there is an opportunity to enact change.

As we embark on this journey of understanding, let us not lose sight of the individuals behind the numbers—the silent warriors who wage a daily battle against cancer with unwavering resolve. Their stories inspire us, their struggles unite us, and their resilience fuels our determination to uncover the mysteries of youth cancer and to advocate tirelessly for awareness and research.

In the chapters that follow, we will delve deeper into the complexities of the youth cancer surge, exploring the myriad factors at play and the urgent need for action. But for now, let us pause to reflect on the courage of those who walk this path, and to reaffirm our commitment to stand beside them in the fight against youth cancer.

Chapter 2

Unveiling the Mystery

In the vast landscape of medicine, where every diagnosis is akin to solving a puzzle, the enigma of youth cancer emerges as a formidable challenge, confounding even the most seasoned experts and researchers. It stands as a complex puzzle, shrouded in mystery, leaving behind a trail of unanswered questions and unexplored terrain.

As we peer into the intricate web of youth cancer, we are confronted with a multitude of perplexities, each more confounding than the last. From the diverse array of cancer types affecting young individuals to the elusive nature of its underlying causes, the enigma of youth cancer presents a formidable obstacle to progress.

For medical professionals and researchers alike, the hurdles posed by youth cancer are numerous. How do we reconcile the paradox of youth—a period traditionally associated with health and vigor—with the harsh reality of a cancer diagnosis? How do we untangle the intricate interplay of genetic predisposition, environmental exposures, and lifestyle factors that contribute to cancer development in young adults? And, most crucially, how do we translate our understanding of these complexities into actionable strategies for prevention, detection, and treatment?

These are the questions that drive our pursuit of knowledge, fueling our determination to unravel the mysteries of youth cancer and to pave the way forward in the battle against this insidious disease. Yet, for every question we manage to answer, countless others linger, serving as a testament to the boundless complexity of the human body and the challenges inherent in our quest for comprehension.

However, amidst the uncertainty, there exists a beacon of hope—a glimmer of light piercing through the darkness of the unknown. With each new revelation, each milestone in research, we edge closer to unlocking the secrets of youth cancer and empowering those affected by it with the knowledge and resources they need to confront the future with bravery and resilience.

As we navigate the uncharted waters of the youth cancer enigma, let us be guided by the stories of those who traverse this path—the silent warriors who meet each day with unwavering resolve and unshakable determination. Their courage serves as an inspiration, their struggles bind us together, and their resilience serves as a reminder that even in the face of adversity, hope endures.

In the chapters that lie ahead, we will delve deeper into the mysteries of youth cancer, exploring the latest research discoveries, addressing pressing questions, and charting the most promising avenues for progress. But for now, let us pause to acknowledge the complexity of the challenge before us and reaffirm our commitment to unraveling the enigma of youth cancer—one breakthrough, one discovery at a time.

Chapter 3

Dissecting Trends

In the intricate tapestry of youth cancer, the threads of causation are woven from a myriad of factors—each playing a role in shaping the landscape of risk and resilience for young adults. As we embark on the journey of dissecting trends, we are confronted with a complex interplay of dietary habits, sedentary lifestyles, environmental toxins, genetics, and birth methods—each contributing to the rise in cancer rates among youth in its own unique way.

At the heart of this web of causation lies the question of lifestyle—a powerful determinant of health and well-being for individuals of all ages. In an era marked by convenience and instant gratification, the choices we make about what we eat, how we move, and how we interact with our environment have profound implications for our long-term health. For young adults, whose habits and behaviors are still taking shape, the consequences of these choices are felt most acutely.

Dietary habits, for instance, play a crucial role in shaping cancer risk among youth. The prevalence of processed foods, high in sugar, salt, and unhealthy fats, has become a ubiquitous feature of modern life—a trend that has been linked to increased cancer incidence among young adults. Similarly, sedentary lifestyles, characterized by prolonged periods of sitting and inactivity, have been shown to contribute to the development of cancer in young people—a sobering reminder of the importance of movement and physical activity in maintaining health and well-being.

But the story of youth cancer is not solely one of lifestyle choices—it is also a tale of environmental exposure and genetic predisposition. In an increasingly industrialized world, young adults are exposed to a staggering array of environmental toxins—from air pollution and water contamination to chemical additives and pesticides—all of which have been implicated in the development of cancer. Likewise, genetic factors play a significant role in shaping cancer risk, with certain hereditary conditions predisposing individuals to a higher likelihood of developing cancer at a young age.

Yet, amidst the complexities of youth cancer causation, there is reason for hope—a glimmer of light in the darkness of uncertainty. For with each new discovery, each breakthrough in research, we inch closer to understanding the intricate interplay of factors that contribute to the rise in cancer rates among youth. And with this understanding comes the power to enact change—to advocate for healthier lifestyles, to push for stricter environmental regulations, and to invest in research that will pave the way for a future free from the burden of youth cancer.

In the chapters that follow, we will delve deeper into the complexities of youth cancer causation, exploring the latest research findings, the most pressing questions, and the most promising avenues for progress. But for now, let us pause to reflect on the challenges before us, and to reaffirm our commitment to uncovering the mysteries of youth cancer—one step, one discovery, at a time.

Chapter 4

Elevating Voices

In the silent corridors of hospitals and the quiet moments of reflection, the voices of young cancer patients, survivors, caregivers, and advocates echo with a resonance that cannot be ignored. These are the voices that speak of courage in the face of adversity, resilience in the midst of uncertainty, and hope in the darkest of times. In Chapter 4, we elevate these voices, sharing their compelling personal narratives and testimonies to provide insight into the lived experiences and challenges faced by those affected by youth cancer.

Each story is a testament to the strength of the human spirit—a reminder that even in the face of unimaginable hardship, there is light to be found. From the young cancer patient bravely facing each day with unwavering resolve to the survivor celebrating the milestones of life with newfound appreciation, each voice offers a unique perspective on the journey through youth cancer.

For the young cancer patient, the diagnosis is often met with shock and disbelief—a sudden interruption to the rhythm of life that was once filled with dreams and aspirations. Yet, amidst the fear and uncertainty, there is a determination to fight—to defy the odds and emerge stronger on the other side.

For the survivor, the journey is one of triumph over adversity—a testament to the power of resilience and the resilience of the human spirit. Each milestone reached is a victory—a testament to the courage and perseverance that carried them through the darkest of days.

For the caregiver, the journey is one of selflessness and sacrifice—a relentless commitment to standing by their loved one's side, offering comfort, support, and unwavering love in the face of unimaginable hardship.

And for the advocate, the journey is one of tireless advocacy and relentless determination—to raise awareness, to push for research, and to fight for a future free from the burden of youth cancer.

In sharing these voices, we hope to shine a light on the lived experiences of those affected by youth cancer—to amplify their stories, to honor their courage, and to inspire others to join the fight. For it is only by coming together, by standing united in our determination to uncover the mysteries of youth cancer and to advocate tirelessly for awareness and research, that we can truly make a difference.

So let us listen, let us learn, and let us be inspired by the voices of those who walk this path—the silent warriors who face each day with unwavering resolve and unyielding determination. Their stories remind us that even in the face of adversity, there is always hope—that even in the darkest of times, there is light to be found.

Chapter 5

Advocating Awareness

In the shadowy corners of society, where fear and misunderstanding reign supreme, the specter of cancer casts a long and formidable shadow—a shadow that often falls heaviest on the shoulders of young adults facing the daunting reality of a cancer diagnosis. In Chapter 5, we confront the societal stigma and misconceptions surrounding cancer in young adults, particularly colorectal cancer, and advocate tirelessly for increased awareness, education, and early detection initiatives to combat the stigma and improve outcomes for young cancer patients.

For too long, cancer—particularly colorectal cancer—has been shrouded in secrecy and shame, its mention met with whispers and avoidance. Yet, the reality is far different from the myths and misconceptions that surround it. Colorectal cancer knows no age, no gender, and no social status—it can strike anyone, at any time, with devastating consequences. And for young adults facing a diagnosis, the stigma and misconceptions surrounding this disease only serve to compound the challenges they already face.

But amidst the darkness, there is reason for hope—a beacon of light in the form of increased awareness, education, and early detection initiatives. By shining a spotlight on the realities of colorectal cancer in young adults, we can dispel the myths and misconceptions that perpetuate the stigma surrounding this disease. By empowering young adults with knowledge and resources, we can improve outcomes and save lives.

It begins with education—raising awareness about the signs and symptoms of colorectal cancer, particularly among young adults who may not be aware of their risk.

It continues with advocacy—pushing for increased screening initiatives and early detection programs to ensure that young adults have access to the care they need, when they need it most. And it culminates with action—taking a stand against the stigma and misconceptions that surround colorectal cancer, and advocating tirelessly for a future free from the burden of this devastating disease.

In the chapters that follow, we will delve deeper into the challenges and opportunities surrounding colorectal cancer in young adults, exploring the latest research findings, the most pressing advocacy efforts, and the most promising avenues for progress. But for now, let us pause to reflect on the importance of advocacy in combating stigma and improving outcomes for young cancer patients, and to reaffirm our commitment to standing united in the fight against colorectal cancer—and all cancers—in young adults.

Chapter 6

Charting Paths to Prevention

In the vast expanse of the battle against cancer, prevention stands as a beacon of hope—a glimmer of light in the darkness of uncertainty. In Chapter 6, we delve into the critical strategies and practical guidance necessary for effective cancer prevention among young adults. Our exploration encompasses not only individual lifestyle modifications and screening recommendations but also delves into the vital role of environmental awareness, community engagement, and policy initiatives in fortifying the defenses against youth cancer.

At the core of cancer prevention lies the power of knowledge—empowering individuals with the information they need to make informed choices about their health and well-being. This empowerment begins with education, where young adults learn about the impact of lifestyle choices on their cancer risk. By adopting healthier habits, such as consuming a balanced diet rich in fruits and vegetables, engaging in regular physical activity, maintaining a healthy weight, and avoiding tobacco and excessive alcohol consumption, young adults can significantly reduce their risk of developing cancer later in life.

However, prevention is not solely an individual endeavor—it thrives within the context of community support and engagement. Communities play a pivotal role in fostering environments that promote health and well-being, from implementing policies that encourage access to nutritious foods and safe spaces for physical activity to supporting initiatives that reduce exposure to environmental toxins and carcinogens. By fostering a culture of wellness and resilience, communities can empower young adults to make healthier choices and navigate the challenges of cancer prevention with confidence.

Screening also plays a crucial role in cancer prevention, allowing for the early detection and treatment of cancer before it has a chance to spread. Young adults are encouraged to follow recommended screening guidelines for various cancers, including breast, cervical, colorectal, and skin cancer, among others. Regular screenings enable healthcare providers to identify cancer at its earliest stages when it is most treatable and curable, offering young adults the best chance for a positive outcome.

Moreover, environmental awareness is paramount in the pursuit of cancer prevention, as exposure to environmental toxins and pollutants can significantly increase the risk of cancer among young adults. By advocating for cleaner air, water, and food, and supporting policies that protect the environment and public health, individuals and communities can reduce their exposure to carcinogens and minimize the risk of cancer in young adults.

In the chapters that follow, we will delve deeper into the strategies and initiatives aimed at preventing youth cancer, exploring the latest research findings, the most effective prevention programs, and the most promising avenues for progress. But for now, let us pause to reflect on the power of prevention in the fight against cancer and to reaffirm our commitment to working together to create a future free from the burden of youth cancer.

Chapter 7

Inspiring Action

In the face of the daunting youth cancer epidemic, there emerges a symphony of resilience, courage, and relentless determination—a testament to the human spirit's unwavering ability to confront adversity with unwavering resolve. In Chapter 7, we immerse ourselves in the stories of individuals and organizations who serve as beacons of hope, tirelessly leading efforts to raise awareness, fund research, and provide support to young cancer patients and survivors. Through their inspiring examples, we not only find solace and encouragement but also discover the power within ourselves to effect change and combat the youth cancer epidemic.

From the humble beginnings of grassroots initiatives to the far-reaching impact of large-scale advocacy campaigns, the landscape of youth cancer activism is as diverse as it is impactful. At its heart are the stories of young cancer survivors who transform their personal battles into powerful platforms for advocacy, using their experiences to illuminate the struggles faced by young adults confronting cancer and inspire hope in those who walk a similar path. Their resilience, courage, and unwavering commitment to making a difference serve as a beacon of light, guiding others through the darkness of uncertainty and fear.

Equally inspiring are the healthcare professionals and researchers who dedicate their lives to advancing the field of youth oncology, tirelessly working to uncover the mysteries of youth cancer and develop innovative treatments that offer hope to young patients and their families. Their groundbreaking research and tireless advocacy for improved patient care drive progress in the fight against youth cancer, offering a glimmer of hope in the face of adversity.

Yet, perhaps most remarkable are the countless organizations—both large and small—that provide invaluable support and resources to young cancer patients and their families, offering a lifeline of assistance and compassion in their time of need. From local cancer support groups to international advocacy organizations, these entities play a vital role in fostering a community of care and support for those affected by youth cancer, offering hope and assistance where it is needed most.

As we immerse ourselves in these stories of courage, compassion, and resilience, let us be inspired to take action in our own communities, to become advocates for change, and to stand in solidarity with those affected by youth cancer. Whether it's volunteering our time, raising funds for research, or simply spreading awareness among our peers, each of us has the power to make a difference in the fight against youth cancer. Let us stand united in our determination to create a future free from the burden of youth cancer—and let us take action today to make that future a reality.

Chapter 8

Pursuing Solutions

In Chapter 8, we embark on a journey of discovery and innovation, exploring the cutting-edge approaches and advancements in cancer research, treatment modalities, and survivorship care that hold the promise of improving outcomes for young cancer patients. Through our exploration, we delve into the intricate tapestry of scientific inquiry and medical innovation, seeking to unravel the mysteries of youth cancer and pave the way for a future free from its devastating grip.

At the forefront of our exploration are the groundbreaking advancements in cancer research that have revolutionized our understanding of the disease and opened new avenues for treatment. From targeted therapies and immunotherapy to precision medicine and genomics, researchers are harnessing the power of innovation to develop more effective and personalized treatments for young cancer patients. Through collaborative efforts and interdisciplinary research, scientists are unraveling the complex genetic and molecular mechanisms driving cancer growth, offering hope for more precise and targeted interventions that spare young patients from the harsh side effects of traditional treatments.

Equally important are the strides being made in survivorship care, as healthcare providers and survivorship advocates work together to address the unique needs and challenges faced by young cancer survivors. From fertility preservation and psychosocial support to long-term monitoring and survivorship clinics, survivorship care programs are evolving to provide comprehensive and holistic care to young cancer patients beyond the completion of their treatment. By addressing the physical, emotional, and social aspects of survivorship, these programs are empowering young cancer survivors to reclaim their lives and thrive beyond cancer.

Yet, perhaps the most compelling aspect of our exploration is the spirit of collaboration and collective action that drives progress in the fight against youth cancer. Across the globe, researchers, healthcare providers, policymakers, and advocates are joining forces to confront the challenges posed by youth cancer and work towards finding solutions. Through collaborative research initiatives, data sharing platforms, and patient advocacy networks, these stakeholders are breaking down silos, fostering innovation, and accelerating progress towards a future where youth cancer is no longer a threat.

As we journey through the realm of cancer research, treatment, and survivorship care, let us be inspired by the progress being made and the potential for change that lies ahead. Let us remain steadfast in our commitment to uncovering the mysteries of youth cancer, advocating tirelessly for awareness and research, and standing in solidarity with young cancer patients and their families. For in our collective efforts lies the power to transform the landscape of youth cancer care and create a future where every young person can live free from the burden of cancer.

Chapter 9

Nurturing Hope

In Chapter 9, we turn our gaze towards the shining beacons of hope amidst the shadows of the youth cancer epidemic, weaving together stories of resilience, courage, and unwavering optimism that illuminate the path forward. With a profound understanding of the challenges faced by young cancer patients and their families, we embark on a journey of inspiration and empowerment, determined to nurture hope in the face of adversity and uncertainty.

As we traverse the landscape of youth cancer, we encounter stories that defy despair and embody the indomitable human spirit. From the young cancer patients who face each day with courage and grace, to the survivors who emerge from the depths of darkness with newfound strength and resilience, their stories serve as a testament to the power of hope in the face of adversity. Through their experiences, we witness the transformative power of optimism, resilience, and unwavering determination to overcome the greatest of obstacles.

Take, for instance, the story of Emily, a vibrant young woman who was diagnosed with leukemia at the age of 21. Despite facing grueling rounds of chemotherapy and a bone marrow transplant, Emily refused to let cancer define her. Instead, she embraced each day with a spirit of hope and optimism, finding joy in the simple moments of life and inspiring those around her with her unwavering positivity. Today, Emily is not just a survivor—she is a beacon of hope for others facing similar battles, reminding us all that even in our darkest moments, hope has the power to light the way forward.

But hope does not exist in isolation—it thrives in the embrace of community, compassion, and unwavering support. As we immerse ourselves in the stories of young cancer patients and survivors, we are reminded of the importance of fostering a culture of hope and optimism in the face of the youth cancer epidemic. Through acts of kindness, empathy, and solidarity, we can uplift and empower those affected by youth cancer, offering them the support and encouragement they need to navigate the challenges of their journey with courage and determination.

Consider the example of the Cancer Hope Foundation, a grassroots organization founded by a group of young cancer survivors with a mission to spread hope and positivity to others facing similar battles. Through their outreach programs, support groups, and survivorship events, the foundation offers a lifeline of hope to young cancer patients and their families, reminding them that they are not alone in their journey. By fostering a sense of community and connection, the Cancer Hope Foundation empowers young cancer patients to face each day with renewed strength and resilience, knowing that they have a network of support behind them every step of the way.

Yet, amidst the trials and tribulations of the youth cancer epidemic, hope remains our most powerful weapon in the fight against despair. It is a beacon of light that guides us through the darkest of times, illuminating the path forward and inspiring us to press on in the face of adversity. As we bear witness to the stories of resilience, courage, and hope that abound in the youth cancer community, let us be inspired to nurture hope in our own lives and the lives of those around us. For in hope lies the power to transcend obstacles, conquer challenges, and create a future where every young person can live free from the burden of cancer.

Chapter 10
Forging a Cancer-Free Tomorrow

In the final chapter of our journey through the landscape of youth cancer, we find ourselves at a pivotal moment—a moment of reflection, inspiration, and unwavering determination to forge a future where youth cancer is but a distant memory. As we stand on the threshold of change, it is imperative that we not only acknowledge the challenges that lie ahead but also embrace the boundless possibilities that await us.

Throughout this book, we have embarked on a profound exploration of youth cancer, delving into its complexities, uncovering its mysteries, and bearing witness to the stories of resilience, courage, and hope that define the human spirit in the face of adversity. From the statistical trends and data that illuminate the scope of the youth cancer epidemic to the personal narratives and testimonies that offer glimpses into the lived experiences of those affected, our journey has been both enlightening and humbling.

As we reflect on the insights gained from our exploration, it becomes clear that the fight against youth cancer is not one that can be waged in isolation. It is a battle that requires the collective efforts of individuals, communities, and organizations united in a shared mission to eradicate this devastating disease. It is a battle that demands compassion, determination, and unwavering resolve—a battle that we must wage together, hand in hand, until every young person is free from the burden of cancer.

But how do we translate our knowledge and insights into meaningful action? How do we take the first step towards creating a future where youth cancer is a thing of the past? The answer lies in the power of advocacy, awareness, and community engagement. It lies in our ability to stand up, speak out, and join the movement for change.

First and foremost, we must advocate tirelessly for increased awareness, education, and research funding to combat youth cancer. We must raise our voices in support of policies and initiatives that prioritize the needs of young cancer patients and survivors, ensuring access to quality care, treatment options, and support services. By amplifying the voices of those affected by youth cancer, we can shine a spotlight on this often-overlooked issue and drive meaningful change at the local, national, and global levels.

Additionally, we must work together to foster a culture of hope and optimism in the face of adversity. We must celebrate the stories of resilience, courage, and perseverance that abound in the youth cancer community, uplifting and empowering those affected by cancer to face each day with renewed strength and determination. Through acts of kindness, empathy, and solidarity, we can create a supportive and nurturing environment where young cancer patients and survivors can thrive, knowing that they are not alone in their journey.

Furthermore, we must equip ourselves with the knowledge and resources needed to take action in the fight against youth cancer. Whether through volunteering with cancer organizations, participating in fundraising events, or advocating for policy change, each one of us has the power to make a difference. By coming together as a collective force for good, we can drive progress, foster innovation, and create a world where youth cancer is no longer a threat.

In closing, I invite you, the reader, to join me in this movement for change. Together, let us stand as beacons of hope, advocates for progress, and champions of a brighter future. Let us commit ourselves to the fight for a cancer-free tomorrow, where every young person can live their lives to the fullest, free from the shadow of cancer. For in our collective efforts lies the power to transform lives, inspire change, and create a world where youth cancer is no more.

Conclusion

As we come to the end of our journey together, I want to emphasize once again the profound importance of understanding, awareness, and action when it comes to addressing the youth cancer enigma. Throughout this book, we've explored the intricate web of challenges that young cancer patients face, from diagnosis to treatment and beyond. We've delved into the statistics, unpacked the data, and listened closely to the voices of those affected by this relentless disease.

But behind every statistic, every data point, and every medical term, there are real people—brave young warriors and their families—who are living this reality every single day. Their stories, their struggles, and their triumphs have touched our hearts and inspired us to keep pushing forward, even when the road ahead seems daunting.

I want to take a moment to express my deepest gratitude to everyone who has contributed to this book—to the researchers who tirelessly search for answers, the healthcare professionals who provide care and support, and the advocates who tirelessly raise awareness and champion the cause of youth cancer prevention and support. But most of all, I want to thank the young warriors themselves—the true heroes of this story—for their resilience, their courage, and their unwavering spirit in the face of unimaginable challenges.

As we close this chapter, I urge each and every one of you, my fellow readers, to carry the lessons learned and the stories shared within these pages with you on your journey forward. Let us continue to raise our voices, to shine a light on the issues that matter, and to stand in solidarity with those who need our support the most. Together, we can make a difference. Together, we can create a world where youth cancer is no longer a threat.

In closing, I want to say thank you—from the bottom of my heart—for joining me on this journey. Your compassion, your dedication, and your unwavering support mean more than words can express. Let us continue to walk this path together, hand in hand, as we strive to build a brighter future for all.

About the Author

Dr. S.J. Bennett is a distinguished medical professional renowned for their oncology expertise and passionate advocacy for cancer research and awareness. With a career spanning decades, Dr. Bennett has dedicated their life to unraveling the complexities of cancer, particularly among young adults, and to spearheading initiatives aimed at improving outcomes for patients and their families.

Throughout their illustrious career, Dr. Bennett has been at the forefront of groundbreaking research, contributing to numerous studies and publications that have advanced our understanding of cancer causation, treatment modalities, and survivorship care. Their tireless efforts have earned them recognition as a leading authority in the field of oncology, with colleagues and peers alike lauding their intellect, compassion, and unwavering commitment to excellence.

Beyond their contributions to academia and research, Dr. Bennett is also a passionate advocate for cancer awareness and prevention. Through public speaking engagements, community outreach programs, and media appearances, they have worked tirelessly to educate the public about the importance of early detection, healthy lifestyle choices, and the latest advancements in cancer care.

As both a clinician and a researcher, Dr. Bennett brings a unique perspective to their work—one informed by firsthand experience with patients and a deep appreciation for the complexities of cancer as both a disease and a human experience. Their empathy, compassion, and dedication to their patients have earned them the respect and admiration of colleagues, patients, and families alike.

In addition to their professional endeavors, Dr. Bennett is also a devoted mentor and educator, guiding the next generation of medical professionals in their pursuit of knowledge and excellence. Their passion for teaching and their commitment to fostering a culture of curiosity and discovery have left an indelible mark on countless students and trainees.

As they continue their mission to unravel the mysteries of cancer and to advocate for those affected by the disease, Dr. Bennett remains steadfast in their belief that with perseverance, collaboration, and a shared commitment to progress, we can overcome the challenges posed by cancer and pave the way for a future free from the burden of disease.